A LIFE
FORGOTTEN

from the eyes of the caregiver

JUDY THOMPSON

Cover Graphic Design by H.D. Bradford

Library of Congress Cataloging-in-Publication Data
Thompson, Judy
A Life Forgotten: From the Eyes of the Caregiver
/ Judy Thompson.

ISBN-13: 978-1494479060

Printed in the United States of America
Published in the United States by Studio 223

A LIFE FORGOTTEN

from the eyes of the caregiver

*To my family and friends, who allowed me
to vent without judgment.*

Preface

This story follows the devastating disease of Alzheimer's from its inception to its inevitable conclusion. This insidious disease silently steals peoples' lives and destroys the beautiful memories we all cherish. Follow me as I struggle with the progression of my husband's disease, fight against the aggression of the disease itself, and discover what the disease takes away.

Memory as we know it – the repository of the details of our lives – disappears under the onslaught of Alzheimer's. From our childhood to our independence, the loss Alzheimer's exacts is devastating. This culprit not only takes away the memory of people and places, but of all things learned throughout life. The loss of memories of where you were yesterday or what you had for supper the evening before is only the tip of the iceberg.

Alzheimer's disease is the mastermind of illnesses. It is secretive in its arrival, but stays forever. It lets you know indirectly, only after it has taken residency in the brain. It moves slowly and deliberately at first and, when this appalling condition has settled in, it eats away at the memory. Then it speeds up. Imagine the affected person losing *all* the things one has learned through life: names, faces, words, objects, the inability to concentrate, the inability to see clearly and the inability to hear or think coherently. The human mind reduced to nothingness. The effects on the sufferer of this disease are well known; the toll it takes on the caregiver, less so.

This book will explore how this sickness changes the patient as well as the caregiver. Perhaps you are in a similar situation. Perhaps you have family or friends going through this. By reading my experiences, I hope you will understand the anxiety felt by both patient and caregiver, the depression as it seeps into each one. Frustration gives way to anger and irritability. Both of these emotions give in to exhaustion. These feelings are understandable and normal. You do not have to go through this alone.

Realize I have no regrets except that my sweetheart is gone. I would do all again and again just to have him back. And believe me when I tell you my husband passed with dignity and with family by his side. I was fortunate enough that the disease, though it did win in the end, did not take away the respectability my husband always had. He was still in control of his bodily functions and proud of whom he was, right up to the end. My family was proud of calling him father, grandfather, uncle, and friend. And, I am blessed to have been his wife of 22 years.

Judy Thompson

Chapter 1

When did it start? Do I really know? I can only explain that the year I begin this is 2007. I am at the beginning of a very difficult period. My husband and I have been married seventeen wonderful years as of the date of these notes. I say wonderful because the times we have spent together have been next to perfect – until now. We are still happy and living our lives together but something is inching its way between us: memory loss.

Is it dementia or Alzheimer's? There's no way of knowing at this stage. I have also been told it could be the beginning of Parkinson's. If you had a choice, which one would you pick? There is no simple comparison; no problem would be the best. Whatever it is, my husband and I will have to deal with it, together.

There is some confusion as to the difference between dementia and Alzheimer's. Simply put, dementia is a symptom, in the same way a fever is a symptom. The cause of that symptom could be any number of things. In dementia's case, it could be something as simple as vitamin deficiencies, which could be reversible. But in the vast majority of the cases, the cause is Alzheimer's. *It* is not reversible, and it is relentless and insidious in its effects on the lives of the sufferer and the surrounding family. And, specially, on the caregiver.

On the date I write this, my husband, John, is seventy-two years old. He's a little overweight. Okay, a little might be understating it. I try to get him to exercise. He's stubborn, though – typical British. Yes, very British. Born in Yorkshire, England in 1935, he was the only child of Harold and Ruth. I believe I should give you a bit of history here. Maybe, by examining this, I can determine how this disease has entered into my husband's brain. Just maybe, I can see what has triggered this condition to reveal itself at this time.

Harold, John's father, was eleven years younger than Ruth and in fairly good health, with the exception of being a smoker.

In 1965, John moved his family – his wife Audrey and three sons – to the United States of America, the land of opportunity. He always wondered if this drastic move was a good idea for his sons. Later, I always tried to reassure him that moving to this new country would always be his greatest accomplishment. It had been a brave and courageous move and opened up a new wealth of opportunity for himself and his sons. He used to tell me all about the move on a regular basis. Maybe he had forgotten that he mentioned this to me several times in our married life, but it was one of those stories that he told and re-told. He recalled with such pride and happiness that this was his most valued accomplishment – bringing his young sons and his bride Audrey to this wonderful country.

John had worked in England with the Jaguar Company and was an expert mechanic. Jaguar sponsored his move to the United States because only a few mechanics were as accomplished as he was. After arriving in the United States, he worked hard to establish himself as a skilled auto mechanic on all automobiles. After much hard work, he made himself such a worthy repair mechanic that he was able to open his own business. He was successful and was able to earn exactly what he needed in order to provide the best for his family. Later, he even had the ability to bring his parents to American soil to share in his success.

John's parents stayed here in this United States for a few years, but did not make it permanent. Ruth being of senior age decided they needed to move back to England where their roots were. His father Harold died at the age of 75 from lung cancer due to smoking. Fortunately, John inherited this nasty habit for only a very short period of time. John realized the ill effects that smoking could have on the body and decided he needed to quit immediately. He did this long before we met and even before he came to America. His mother, Ruth, lived to be eighty-nine and passed away from natural causes in England as well.

I noticed that John related a lot to his father and not as much to his mother. He would often tell me he was worried about a particular birthday – his seventy-fifth. He felt he may not have the luxury to see it, being that his dad's life ended at that age. John always felt that his would more than likely end around the same time.

What makes someone try and predict their own demise? Could it be fear, dementia, or is it just something everyone does? It was certainly not genes. His mother, Ruth, lived to a ripe old age; those genes were also moving around in John's body. Are we as human beings so negative, or are we predestined to think that we will die at the same age as our parents? We must stop those thoughts and believe that we can extend our lives past the age of our parents. In today's world, age of retirement alone shows our life expectancy is getting a lot longer.

So, John came to the United States with his wife Audrey and his three sons. So where do I fit in the picture, you might ask?

Let me explain who I am. I am John's second wife. We met in a support group after we both lost our spouses. John's wife of 34 years, Audrey, passed away from the devastating disease of pancreatic cancer. Her health was fine and their lifestyle was comfortable until this disease took her from John.

My first husband died of cancer as well, only it was melanoma. John and I became good friends after we met in the support group and soon, a stronger friendship developed. We had so much in common and were able to share our grief as well as our road to adjusting to our loss. We married three years later and that is how I came into this picture.

We continued to grow closer and closer sharing our love and our grief. John tells me all the time how much he loves me, and it feels so wonderful. He tells me I am beautiful. I savor the feeling and keep telling him to get new glasses, or to not be silly, but John keeps telling me that he has been blessed with two of the most wonderful women he has ever known. Of course I loved it. Now, I worry about my husband remembering my name.

He understands that he has a lot of memory loss, mostly short term. Remember here that his memory of *his* memory loss will also wane. We got some help from the doctor who tested his memory over a fifteen-minute period. It is such an easy test, but one that actually shows loss of memory. The doctor gave three words to my husband and asked him to remember them. The doctor then left the room and returned in about five minutes and proceeded to examine John, listening to his heart, feeling his stomach, listening to his chest and at his back to be sure his lungs are clear. Checking eyes, ears, nose, throat, plus the other natural things that a doctor checks. After about twenty minutes of time have passed, the doctor asked John what the three words were that he had asked John to remember. No luck; the words were gone from his mind.

People deal with memory loss in different ways. How does John deal with it? Quite often, he would joke with me but I did *not* find it to be humorous. He would always come back with, "What's your name, anyway?" Oh how I hated that – it made me wonder if he really had forgotten my name. But I could not imagine what was going on in his mind. For John to know that something was taking away his very existence must have been terrifying. Sometimes, he was sad and weepy. The depression was moving in. Again, are these the beginnings of dementia or Alzheimer's, or is it just the fear of growing older? He told me each day how he felt. I would ask, "How do you feel today?" He answered me with, "I feel lousy".

I needed to pinpoint the problem for the doctor – "lousy" just doesn't cut it. I tried to have him describe what he felt so we could relay these symptoms to the doctor and can get the answers we needed. I really needed him to express deeply what he was feeling so I could help him as we explain these things to our primary physician. If I understood his feelings, I would be better equipped to explain them to the doctor, and maybe relieve some of the pain he is feeling.

We will be going to a neurologist in August and will be talking to him to find out if it could be Parkinson's that is causing the memory loss. I have heard that, in addition to the shaking and anxiety problems, Parkinson's can cause memory loss as well. No one can at this time diagnose Alzheimer's accurately until death, and hopefully we are far from that.

I, like a lot of others that may be dealing with memory loss, feel I can handle the loss of his memory. I know I can remember for both of us. Oh, how I wish it were that easy! I have a fine memory, but it is that which he cannot remember that is so frustrating.

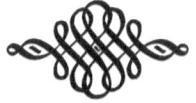

Chapter 2

John tells me, in his words, "I feel dizzy, lightheaded, and lethargic, almost as if something has drained every bit of my energy. I feel yucky."

It is the fall of 2007 and my wonderful husband got laid off from his courier job at ReMax. I guess if I had to put a date on it I would have to say that September 2007 was the beginning. Once John got laid off, it seemed our life began to change. The changes, as I write this, are visible only to me. They are very subtle, but noticeable to me. He can control himself enough that others may not notice.

The end of one chapter became the beginning of another. John's life was now changing. He no longer needed to work – or was it work no longer needed him? One of our sons told him, "At your age, it's about time you retired and enjoyed life. Lounge around, feel the sunlight, start a garden. Take some short trips with Mom, or just relish in your accomplishments."

Sounds like a great idea, right? Until you check the year: 2007. This year began the major downturn in the economy. The price of real estate was crashing down around us and his courier position was no longer viable. There was no money coming in. It was definitely a new beginning – just one we hadn't planned for.

It's easy to say, "take trips," but money was and still is a big factor in whether or not trips are in the future. Unfortunately, the trips we took were from one doctor to another.

The first doctor was the primary physician in late 2007. The doctor was great; based on the symptoms, he suggested that we should see a cardiac specialist to check the symptoms of John's heart racing, and the other symptoms of palpitations, dizziness, breathlessness and lightheadedness. Even the hands shaking would be checked. We made the appointment for early in 2008.

We trotted off to the cardiac specialist. For the next several months, we were so busy with our trips to the cardiologist you would have thought we were preparing for our college finals in cardiology. Through all the testing – whether from blood, or angioplasty – we were able to rule out serious heart problems. The cardiologist said that his heart was strong and healthy.

"But, to be sure, let's do one more test," he said.

John was still having the palpitations in his heart and still felt pretty lousy. The doctors wanted to conduct a stress test. A heart monitor was placed on my husband, which he would wear for 24 hours. I had to push a button each time he told me that he felt the heart racing or the palpitations. To say the least, it was interesting. It was an experiment, a beginning – the foundation for our search.

I wanted to fix this problem for John, to bring back my sweet husband. It would be so nice to hear him say, "Gee, I feel good today."

After returning the monitor to the doctor so he could analyze the results, the doctor found atrial fibrillations.

Wow, we found something, I thought. *Is this what has been wrong with my husband?*

Finally, there was a possible cause for the symptoms. But was it right?

On to medication. Diagnosis in hand, the doctor prescribed medication. Several weeks later, after the medicine was being administered, the symptoms still did not go away. We were left at home to continue trying to decipher what was happening.

Oh, yes, things were happening to John – unexplainable things. Naturally, these trips to doctors' offices took weeks and months. Between running physical stress tests, the series of machine tests, and a steady regimen of blood tests, the days just floated by. More medicine, more time to see if the medicine was working, more checking for negative side effects.

The days and months flew past. We were certainly busy. Before I knew it, more symptoms appeared. Were they the same as what John had been experiencing, or were they the ones that he was experiencing with his memory loss?

The frustration of his memory loss was taking a toll on me. Exasperated I would plug along every day as best I could, trying not to be annoyed. I would repeat myself numerous times and also explain whatever our daily activities were and why we had to do them. Was anything connected?

They were exasperating days, weepy days. Sometimes I would be angry, but I really had to be careful. If I raised my voice – and you will if you deal with this – my husband would become extremely anxious and shaky. I tried to deal with it as best as I could, and we plugged along.

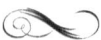

We look to physicians as our healers, put them on pedestals and want them to do God's work. Sometimes, I think we attribute to them supernatural powers. We tell them symptoms, and want results. But doctors are only human. Still, we get frustrated and expect all the answers, if not at least the cure.

Months went by and John's hands were still shaking. Accompanying this was the lightheadedness, the dizziness, the lethargic attitude, the tears. His condition may have not been contagious, but I felt lousy as well.

"I need to see the Doctor. I haven't been telling you, but I have not felt good for sometime now," John told me every few days.

"Excuse me? What did you say? You did not tell me? Are you joking? We've been to three doctors so far," I reminded him.

John must have forgotten that he told me daily how awful he felt. I tried to let it roll off my back. It's not a big deal, I told myself. We all forget.

We went back to the cardiac doctor. At the time, I thought it must be his heart. The doctor decided that we needed to check John's heart for one full week on a special monitor. The device would get hooked up and remain on 24/7 unless he had to shower.

We got home, and I got to work hooking him up to the machine. The photo in the instructions showed exactly where to place the prongs and hook up the wiring. I did a great job.

Every time John felt his heart race, he would press a button and record the heart beats. Then, I would call the number written on the monitor and hold the recorder to the speaker on the phone and record it directly with the nurses at the receiving end of the phone.

The results? Atrial Fibrillations, again. The doctor advised John to continue on his prescribed medications. We were back to square one.

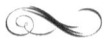

More office visits. Our life was becoming one unending parade of medical providers. Our primary doctor and I talked and decided that John should add an antidepressant to his daily regimen. So many pills! Cholesterol medication, an aspirin a day, an antidepressant, and Coumadin, Namenda, and Aricept. And we still needed to find out why his hands were shaking.

That meant more doctors. Early in 2009, we went to another neurologist to check on the hand shaking that was bothering John. I'd always seen a lot of elderly folks with shaking hands, but never thought much of it. I did not really see the struggle that John expressed. But then again, it was not happening to me.

This new doctor asked John to walk barefooted so he could see how his balance was. He asked John to hold out his hands so he could see the tremors that John was suffering. Though the cause was still undetermined, the doctor ruled out Parkinson's.

The doctor then asked about the new medicines that John was taking. I had brought the list of medications and the only one that was a fairly new drug was

Mididrine. This medicine had been added, as we were looking for anything to control the dizziness John was experiencing daily. After multiple tests, the doctor discovered that John had a drop in blood pressure after going from a sitting position to a standing position. This was explained as A-Fib, and the Mididrine prescription was continued to relieve this situation.

This Midirine did not help his physical or emotional symptoms. Perhaps, in looking for the cause of the lethargy and the anxiety he had been feeling as well as the dizziness, the A-Fib was discovered totally by accident. We were lucky it was discovered, and it helped this other condition. The condition of his sitting and standing and the fast change in his blood pressure was resolved by this medication. We were still in search of answers to the problem he has been suffering with for such a long time.

John had been in discomfort since September, 2007. Again, I begged to anyone that would listen, "Help!"

We visited the neurologist again. He put John on an anti-anxiety drug called Clonazepam. He did not want to add too much to John's current array of medications, which is understandable. Off we went to fill the prescription. It was just one more pill, one more line on his list of medications. The problem, sadly, remained the same.

John was impatient. "Give it a chance to work," I said. My gosh, we just added this new pill to the regimen and we have to see if it is going to work. It will take a while before it goes into his system, I told him.

After about two weeks of this new medication, my husband broke out with a red rash on his chest. He was terribly itchy. After talking with the doctor, I stopped the pill and within a week the rash disappeared. We, of course discontinued this medication.

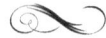

Months went by. There was no change. We went back to see our primary physician. He was so easy to talk to and, of course, we totally trusted him. He was one doctor that knew us. We were not just a number in his practice; there are people that he knew by name and he also knew our children, who he has been taking care of for thirteen years. We entrusted this man to help us in our need, so off we went to make an appointment to see him.

At his office, I asked myself, "What do we say this time?" It seems like he's run every test there is. I asked if there was any test that he had forgotten. He told us that maybe we better just relax and see how things go for the next couple of months; all the results so far were showing that everything was normal.

So, we went home and enjoyed what life had to offer. Things went along as normal as can be and we enjoyed our lives. Of course, the exception was my husband getting up every morning and feeling lousy. Yep, things were normal, alright. I told him, "you feel like crap, but you're okay. Everything is fine with your heart and any problems you feel are really not physical."

Is this what normal is supposed to be? Was there really pain or was this psychosomatic? The only pain was in the mind, according to the tests. How is one told that the pain being felt is not real? That is so unrealistic. So, we proceeded with what we thought was a normal life. Does that mean our thoughts and feelings are abnormal?

My question, of course, was, "What's normal?" When I turn seventy-four or seventy-five, am I going to feel lousy? That doesn't seem right. I was a healthy sixty-four year-old woman feeling like I was turning fifty-five, while my husband was seventy-four going on eighty-five.

Something was not right. That ten-year difference was turning into twenty with neither of us doing anything different.

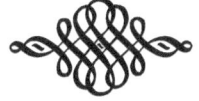

Chapter 3

2010 arrived, and things only got worse. We needed to expand our medical investigation. This problem was escalating and we needed answers. His memory was getting worse, but he was still able to conceal it in front of people. I noticed that he was forgetting some words, calling things he sees by different names.

The doctor suggested that John have an MRI to see what his brain looked like. I thought this was a good idea, so off we went to the imaging center.

The results revealed that John had many spaces within the walls of the brain, showing evidence of dementia, or even Alzheimer's. So, which was it and what is the difference? The doctor explained that dementia can be caused by any number of things, including Alzheimer's. There was no way of knowing what the cause was. But at least, we knew where the memory loss was coming from.

But, we were still in search of the source of the irritation and pain. Most of the answers we were seeking were that everyone with Alzheimer's – if indeed that's what it was – reacts differently. Each person has different symptoms and different reactions. But so far no documentation has been discovered or written that says one could feel pain. The disease itself is one that can react differently on each person, but to cause pain has never been acknowledged.

It is important to remember that we still loved each other and that we were living a great, happy life and sharing each moment of each day with all the ups and downs that went with life. We would sit and chat and reminisce. During these times, everything was awesome and we were fine. During these times, we forgot about the memory problems. We just took everything day-by-day. We talked about anything and everything. We watched the dolphins swim by our villa and enjoyed the gorgeous water views and the boats going by. The serenity makes one slow down and just appreciate the small bits of life that normally fly by.

Nevertheless, there were always reminders of the thief stealing John's memories. For example, sitting on the porch, watching the bay, John said, "A really big fish just came out of the water and it was amazing."

It was a dolphin. He had forgotten the word "dolphin". It was almost as if he had seen one for the first time.

Chapter 4

Several months passed. I was at my wits end. John still felt poorly. In spring of 2009, his seventy-fourth birthday neared. His family would be swooping in soon to celebrate. We were all looking forward to this exciting time.

John was elated that his family came to see him. He felt lucky that he brought his sons to America those many years ago so that they too could have the freedom that he has so enjoyed through the years. Oh, how happy he was! And he wanted his boys to know the happiness he felt.

Was his memory failing? Oh no, not that day.

The first night of the family visit, he felt fine and he knew all that was going on around him. He told me that he remembered that day in the cold of winter when Audrey and their three sons arrived at Logan Airport in 1965. There he was in Boston, with only a name and address of someone he was supposed to meet who would give him the opportunity that he so desired. He recounted how he was willing to work hard for his employer so that the opportunity to enjoy the American way would be his. And he accomplished that dream. That day, he remembered. That day, he knew how blessed he was.

That first night visiting with family, we went to bed at 1:00 AM – dreadfully late for both of us. John was very happy to be with his sons and the entire family.

The following day, John spoke to me and told me that he often thought that he should NOT have made that powerful decision to come to the states. I calmed him, knowing that the decision was by far the best and most life-changing one that he could have ever have made. Then, he told me he thanked God daily for stepping in to guide him in the most traumatic decision of his life. Oddly enough, he was not a religious man. Beyond any doubt, he made the best and most paramount decision of his life. Anything else would be so insignificant it would never need mentioning here.

That day, I felt good and things were what they were supposed to be. I listened to John's heart, took his blood pressure, and asked all sorts of questions, and had come to the conclusion that everything was the same as it had been for a while so we could go about the day with our company.

The following day was the big day. The family all gathered for the celebration of John's birthday. We were all very excited. There were so many of us. There was Dave, his oldest son with his wife and their two children, and Paul, his middle son with his wife and their two children and John's youngest son, Barry. Also there were our family which includes my son, Jonathan and his wife and their three children and my daughter, Katie, with her boyfriend. My daughter-in-law and my son live close by and see us often; we have become close to my daughter-in-law's family, who also came over to help us celebrate this milestone of a birthday. This included six more people to our festivities. This day, however, John felt blue when his family arrived. Why? They were only here for such a short time and would be going home in four days. It was truly not the time to think about that on their arrival. "Chill out and enjoy their visit, we can always be sad in a few days," I told him.

That evening was a totally different story. John's life had dramatically changed: from the quiet, serene life of sitting daily playing on his computer while I worked, to a hectic day cooking and making sure everyone had everything they needed. We had lots of people and commotion, as well as an incredible amount of noise. Was it the noise factor that set him off, or the people enjoying the pool during a fabulously warm day when fun was definitely on the agenda? Whatever it was, it did a job on John.

John had a reaction to the crowd of people sharing our home. Though our company was all family, his nervousness due to noise and the many people around caused him to sweat and shake. He was afraid. No one seemed to pick up on it, but I could recognize it: a panic attack had taken over his body.

That night, he decided to retire to bed at 7:30 pm. It was extremely early, but he needed to leave behind the noise, the group, and all the commotion, which I believe was a contributing factor in this panic attack.

The next morning all was calm, and John didn't even remember going to bed early. It was no big deal.

So what? I thought – totally unimportant. He was just enjoying his son's visit and having the entire family around him.

But then, during the day, John started to weep. "I am so happy that I made that move to America," he said. "I only hope my boys realize what an incredible choice I made for them over 40 years ago," he went on. And the tears flowed.

At this, his sons gathered around to give him the comfort he needed. They reassured him that his decision to come to the United States was one that opened lots of doors to each of them. John felt better after their assurance. Here, it seemed he had lost his confidence and his security.

The day came when the family had to return back to Massachusetts to their own lives and families. That day, I would deal with the sadness and the tears. Together, we would be fine.

On the way home from the airport John and I talked about the visit, and the happiness it brought and sadness it left. But we moved on and found the solace back at home that we had missed for the past few days.

It was too quiet.

"Can we bring them back?" he asked.

I guess we would have to wait until the next birthday.

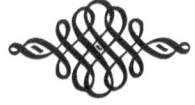

Chapter 5

Life calmed down and the tears subsided. Our life remained sedentary and quiet and things progressed toward another year. I continued to work part time and as many hours as I was allowed. We really needed the money, and I was still trying to discover the problems eating away at my husband.

Sometimes, I was concerned that the feelings of despair were caused by the loss of his job as a courier. Once again, his days began with the feelings of lethargic emotions, dizziness and total discomfort. How could this be memory loss? It seemed more physical than mental.

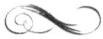

A new situation arose that had no explanation. John could not get out of bed to go to the bathroom. Somehow, he was unable to walk. It was bizarre. *What happened, and was it permanent?* I asked myself.

Off we went to the hospital, where a new series of tests began. John said his pain was a ten on a scale of one to ten, with ten being the highest level. Many extra blood tests were taken but nothing out of order was found. A day or two later, all was fine. His ability to walk returned. Alzheimer's is different for everyone – the remark I hear continuously with each doctor visit.

Chapter 6

The Christmas season was around the corner and – surprise, surprise – we had a guest visit us from Massachusetts: John's youngest son, Barry. We were so happy to see him, even if it was only for three days. It always made John happy to see his children. During this visit, John was very lucid, though there certainly was evidence of memory loss.

Poor John, though he was very happy to see his son, he asked me where Barry would be staying and I explained that Barry would be staying in our spare bedroom. John said he didn't realize we had an extra bedroom. In the mornings, Barry was such an early riser, John would awaken and be concerned about the slight noises we heard in the kitchen and then the awesome aroma of bacon cooking. "Who is in our house" John would whisper to me, I would remind him that Barry was our guest for a few days.

A word about hygiene. I had to keep suggesting that John take a shower. He would cry and moan that he just did not have the energy. To my mind, this was just one more symptom of this oncoming disease.

John's lack of energy was a constant struggle. He told me his head ached – not a headache, but a pain around his eyes at the bridge of his nose. He was frequently cold and wanted to sleep and sleep some more. His eyesight seemed to be failing and he needed new glasses. He cried very easily, mostly because he understood that something was taking his memories and taking his ability to think.

One day, I tried to convince him to go out for a short walk. I can push him in his wheelchair, but I believe his pride had gotten the best of him and he refused to go. He told me his entire body was quivering inside and he did not want to deal with this feeling; he just wanted it to go away. The poor dear was so tired of feeling lousy.

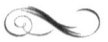

It's Christmas, 2009 and we were going to our son's house with our daughter and her boyfriend. We were looking forward to seeing the grandchildren open their gifts and enjoy a family meal with everyone there. Well, the children opened their gifts and even John was smiling like everything was fine. It was so gratifying for me to see him actually laugh and smile and seem to relax. I was afraid to talk to him for fear he may remember that he feels lousy.

It was a day I wanted to keep secure in the happiness that surrounded it. But, as we enjoyed the meal and the excitement died down and everyone was sitting and relaxing and chatting, I could see that my sweet husband was not feeling like himself. He wanted to go home early. We did. It was a good holiday, for the most part. But my Christmas wish was that I could find something that would make John feel like himself again, or at least calm and without pain.

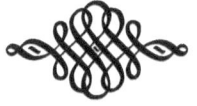

Chapter 7

Several months have gone by since my last writing, as things are progressing slowly. It's a new year, 2010. Thank the good Lord for that anyway.

Will this be a year that we will find the culprit that is stealing my husband's smile, his laugh, his happy-go-lucky life? Please let this be the year that my sweet husband will find the source of the pain and we can eliminate it with the medications that the doctors will prescribe.

Life with my sweet husband was changing forever. The memory loss was explained but the pain continued. He was still taking Aricept and Namenda to help slow the progress of the Alzheimer's.

I could only wish for my husband's brain to stay intact, but the disease was taking control. His memory, which held so many fun times – the laughter, the knowledge, the lives he had touched, the places we had traveled and all the people we had known – was evaporating like a puddle in the sun.

Many times we talked and I told him that I could take care of any physical problems that he had, but I could not control or take care of his mind. That was the part that I had no control over. I could cook and see to it that he ate properly. I could help him exercise, go for walks with him, insist on him showering, make certain he took his medicine, but I could not control his thoughts. I could not control his memory. He could recall the past for now, but the present continued to elude him.

Alzheimer's is a slowly progressing illness that has little outward physical signs. The normal symptoms are so subtle one would barely notice. The "where did I leave my keys" is just the smallest part. The caregiver will notice far more changes than those who are around less frequently. The caregiver will also find frustration in not just the everyday memory losses, but also the changes in the lifestyle. The relationship and the challenges of everyday life begin to mount up. Things become ever so strange. I found not only the memory crumbles, but the sufferer's energy collapses with it. The fact is the patient does not want to move or do anything. Just let them sit and stare into space.

Once, we had a normal routine. But that is no more. Just emptying the trash was a thing of the past. It is not for any other reason except that my poor dear husband had forgotten where to take the trash. Yes, his memory fails him, but yet he could still feel the emotion of embarrassment. How so?

We as caregivers find the understanding of how to do something so routine and simple so basic that we do not think twice about it. But this simple understanding will elude the patient.

John is aware of his memory loss. It is *I* who must remember that he has memory loss. Doing routine things in the house as well as traveling about, taking care of errands and just chatting can become a challenge for the *caregiver*.

I was living a normal existence and I had to remember than John could not remember. That was my challenge. Life moves along and there are times when things appear normal, so I would forget that my husband had memory loss.

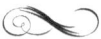

How do we think of memory loss? Do we forget what movie we saw last week, or what we had for supper last night, or the last vacation we took? Oh, no, that's not it; that would be too easy to figure out. Read on and I will show what else memory loss has done.

John's hygiene habits have changed dramatically. He doesn't shower daily as was his normal routine. I plead with him to take a shower and shave to no avail. He has put his electric shaver next to his chair for convenience, but still can't figure out what to do with it, so shaving has become a rare occurrence. I have now become the Barber who cuts his hair and gives him a hot shave. His manicurist is also a new responsibility added to my list.

Now, about those showers... I beg him to take a shower. "Why?" he asks. "I am not going anywhere and I haven't done anything so obviously I am not dirty."

I ask myself how did the thinking change so drastically?

Early in life we learn we must shower regularly to get clean, get the sweat, the dust and dirt off our bodies on a daily basis. Working can create more sweat and daily dirt, but just doing nothing doesn't shut our bodies down so that we don't perspire, we continue to secrete fluids from our pores that need to be cleaned in order to prevent diseases from attacking us.

Well, I would talk to John about his showers and he would explain to me that it took too much energy to take a shower. It was energy he didn't have.

"I haven't the strength to get up and get in the shower. It just takes too much out of me," he told me. Then, another day he would comment that he was too afraid to take a shower. He felt that he would slip and fall and break a bone. He was just too tired and would postpone the shower to another time. But of course, "another time" just never came.

I need to change this. He has to shower. We sleep in the same bed and I want him to be clean. I have an idea: we will shower together.

It worked.

Our first shower together in 19 years. Surely it was different – nothing like the good old days. Well, that's okay. This time it is strictly for cleanliness. John sits on a shower chair while I soap him and wash his hair. I rinse us both and now, the finale. I must get him up on his feet – on which he is very weak – so that I can dry him off and get him dressed and back in his comfy chair. John begins to use me to help him rise. I am wet and slippery, as is he.

He uses my arms, which are wet, and begins to pull himself up. I am slipping and he is slipping. *Oh my God, please don't let us fall*, I pray. I sit him back down and get out of the shower alone and get two towels out one for John and one for me. He tries to dry himself while in the shower as I am drying myself off. I finally get him out of the shower where I continue to dry him off carefully.

He is a rather large person and I don't want him to get any rashes so I must be particularly careful to dry off every crevice and powder him down so that no dampness creates friction due to lack of movement. We make it. He is clean and safe and back in his easy chair. I am thoroughly exhausted. What a job.

I get him to shower with me at least twice a week. After that first one, it is not easy to convince him to take a shower with me. But it is something I push him on so that he gets clean and I can dress him in clean clothes. He insists that unless he is going out – which is nearly never – he does not need a shower or need to change his clothes from his pajamas. I try to convince him that a shower and clean clothes will make him feel so much better.

This goes on for several months, taking its toll on me. I am pretty resourceful, but this is really becoming a very enormous task. I am not only afraid for my husband falling and pulling down our glass shower doors on both of us, but I am afraid for myself as well. After all, without me, who will take care of my husband?

I need to give some thought as to what is my next step in John's care. I am doing all this, maintaining a part time job and running all the errands. I don't mind. He is such a great man and we have had such a great relationship. I just wish he wasn't in pain. The fluttering between his eyes, just above his nose, what is it from? How can we get rid of it? I never thought Alzheimer's' caused pain.

The rubbing, the friction, the constant touching, picking his face with anything he can get his hands on is another part of the disease. He grabs a knife, scissors, tweezers, fingernail file – even a toothpick – to scratch off anything he feels does not belong on his skin.

His face between his eyes is raw with blood and scabs. His arms are scratched and bloody, his ears are scratched and bloody. He has even attacked his legs where he can reach. This is all a part of the disease, I am told. I am also reminded that each person living with the disease has different symptoms. No two people are alike. My sheets are bloody; his pillowcase has to be changed at least 3 times in a week. His shirts are bloody and there is even blood on his easy chair. I try to keep it covered, but that appears to be useless.

Of course, we went to a dermatologist to see if there was a cause for the picking. The answer, yes; keep your hands off your face and any scabs that may form, the dermatologist said. How do we keep scabs from forming on these cuts? Since most of his picking is on his face the doctor told me to keep Vaseline on the injury so that it doesn't dry and cause a scab.

Now, as a ritual, John puts Vaseline over his entire face and neck. This works for a while, until he forgets about it. I am almost glad he forgets, as now he looks like a greasy person. His clothes are stained with the oil from the Vaseline and the pillowcases are hopeless. Another new habit is forming as well. He takes a tissue and rips it into tiny strips and rolls it between his fingers as if making something.

Every day, I deal with his forgetfulness. Earlier this week, I was getting some clean towels out of the linen closet when I found some of my missing underwear in there. Why? John could not remember where it was supposed to go. He was helping me with the laundry, and that was as good as any other place to leave it evidently. Lucky for me my husband still tries to do the laundry. Seem unusual, of course, but that is a habit he has been doing for a number of years. It has been a great help over the years. But how much longer can he do this? Only the Lord can know the answer to that.

I continue to let him do the laundry, though it has not been without some questions or problems. One day, I picked up a white towel and found this blue area on the towel and when I touched it, it appeared to be thick and somewhat sticky. I thought it was some type of bluing, but to my dismay it was not. Then, I thought it was some sort of softener, but again to my dismay it was not. Next I took the section of the towel and put it under running hot water and lots of soap bubbles appeared proving to me that it was liquid laundry soap which was left on the clothes, and towels, as well as most of our personal items. Was this an error on my husband's part, or did something go wrong with the washing machine? I would never know.

Oh well, lets go on to the next situation. My love is still doing the laundry and things appear to be fine. Something I will deal with at a later time, for now I am lucky to have my laundry taken care of by my spouse.

Chapter 8

Illness strikes our house! This time, the caregiver (me) gets sick. Oh yes, that's me. I get this horrendous pain in my lower left side, thinking oh my God, I have a problem with my ovary. I am in my mid sixties and hopefully I do not have any ovary problems.

Well, it gets so bad I decide to go to the emergency room at the local hospital. I wake John at 4:00 AM and tell him I am going to the hospital emergency room with or without him. As groggy as he was, he did not want to let me go alone. So off to the local hospital we go.

I get admitted and spend the next six days hospitalized and drugged beyond belief. It turned out to be diverticulitis. Hospital staff got it under control. But my husband – now that is another story, as he is home alone!

Here I am under care and he is home on his own. Talk about stress and worry, it did not disappear but multiplied. What the heck was he doing all alone? Was he going to be okay?

Thank God our sons were concerned enough to call him daily to see if he was okay. He was still able to pick up the grandchildren after their release from school. He really enjoys that part of the day as he feels once again needed and feels that he is worth something.

While hospitalized, I talk to him daily, though with the drugs I am subjected to it is a wonder he is able to understand what I am saying. All goes well with my treatment, but all does not go well with John, who seems to daily deteriorate because I am not there to take care of every need.

On my second to last day at the facility, John is on the phone with me but is too ill to come see me. What? This totally does not make sense to me. What is he saying? He said he does not feel well and does not think that he can come visit me. I am now very worried.

Is he sick, or is it just the fact that I am unable to care for his daily needs? Is he taking his daily meds? I am sure that those are being avoided as he is not sure what he should take. If I think back to just prior to my hospitalization, I am sure that the meds that I put in containers for him had run out and that I did not have the time to replenish his supply for the following two weeks.

I hadn't planned for my illness – how could I? I guess the kids of today would say, "my bad." Well, I am sorry, but I am only one person and can only do what I am able to do. If I had known that I was going to be sick and out of commission, I would have set up his medication ahead of time.

At last, I was released from the hospital. John came by to pick me up, but he was not himself. What happened to him? I cannot figure this out. He gets to the hospital but, though I know he is glad I am coming home, he is lethargic and moving very slowly. We drive home without incident.

I am home and things appear to be normal. John does not feel well. He is sad and feeling sickly. Today is Monday night. We go to bed, and I hope that tomorrow will be a better day.

I am sure he has not taken his medication as prescribed for him. Perhaps that was the reason he is feeling so out of sorts. That must be the answer.

The day after I got home from the hospital, things are okay for me but I see my husband not feeling well. I do wish I could do something to help him. Again, it is the same thing. He gets up and feels lousy. What can I do to help him? Okay, I know my husband has memory problems, dementia, or Alzheimer's, but why is he in pain? This is what I want to help. Is loss of memory physically painful? I wouldn't have thought that at all. Again I am reminded that each person suffering with this disease reacts differently.

I am still working part time to help us with our financial problems. Leaving John, even for just a few hours three days a week can present problems for him and for me. I know that he is okay and can keep himself company by playing solitaire on his computer. It amazes me that he can still remember how to play this game our grandson, John James, taught him a year earlier. But somehow, he manages. Another of Alzheimer's mysteries.

Working and caregiving is a challenge. John needs to eat and will not make himself lunch, so I make it for him and leave it in the refrigerator for him. I leave the house fairly early, so he must make himself tea and breakfast in the morning.

I need to put his medication on the kitchen table for him to take when he eats his breakfast. I used to leave it on the kitchen counter so that when I went to work, he would remember to take his meds when he made his tea in the morning.

I stopped doing that when he took my medication in error. I guess it was my fault, but I had not had a problem up to this point. One day, I had set out our medications on the counter, mine by the refrigerator and his on the stove and John got up before I went to work.

He had come into the front bedroom that I used as an office to say good morning. I looked at him and asked "Why are you up so early?" Just to say hi, he said. How sweet. I finished my tea, which was my normal routine before my departing for work, and went to take my medication. I poured myself a glass of orange juice and flipped the pills into my mouth, when all of a sudden I spit them out into my hand realizing that I do not take any pink pills. A couple of the pills I do take though are blue and I did not remember popping any blue pills into my mouth.

Once I spit them out I realized that they were my husband's. It dawned on me that my husband had taken *my* medications. When they tell you do not give your medicine to someone else, I understand a little bit better. My medication is for high blood pressure and my husband takes medication for low blood pressure. I hesitate to think what would happen to either of us if both of us had taken the wrong pills. My blood pressure runs high and I am prescribed three blood pressure pills to lower it while John's meds are the opposite. Had I digested them, I could have gone into some sort of wildly high blood pressure, which could have resulted in a stroke. Since John's pressure is low and my pills would lower his even more, I was not sure what I should do. My immediate thoughts were that my husband would be extremely tired and lethargic and probably sleep all day.

Luckily, it was a short day at work and I came home early about five hours after he took my medication. I thought he would be pretty tired and indolent due to the lowering of his blood pressure, which was already low to start with. He seemed to be fine, though.

It was time for John to pick up our grandchildren from school. He went out to his vehicle and I happened to go outside with him, but stopped to say hello to a neighbor.

John called me over. He was getting sick, and as I approached, he began to projectile vomit. Obviously, he wasn't driving anywhere. I told him to go back into the house and sit down and relax. I would pick up the children. On my way to the school I called our son; he said he would get the children. I turned around and hurried back home to check on John.

He was fine, like nothing had happened. Just sitting in his recliner and playing his solitaire game on his computer.

The next day, he did not get out of bed. He was really despondent and depressed. Could it be the after-effect of my medication?

I called a nurse friend and she explained that it was unusual for the discomfort of the wrong meds to last this long, but it could still happen. She advised for him to drink plenty of fluids, especially water and lay down with his legs higher than his heart. I had him do just that for one day, and he seemed to feel slightly better.

On the third day after taking my medication I expected him to feel like his old self again but he was even more lethargic and slept for all but two hours of the day. Thank goodness that on the fourth day, he was back to his wakeful self. He felt normal, which is to say, lousy. Of course, that has been the new normal for quite some time now.

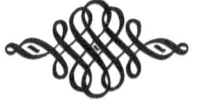

Chapter 9

It was the suggestion of our doctor to get a service dog for John. I explained I live in a 55+ community that did not allow pets. The Doctor said a dog would be beneficial to John's quality of life, and if I got a service animal the Condo Association would have to allow it. So off I went with the prescription for a service dog for my husband. I presented it to the President of our Association who asked that I get two more prescriptions. I contacted the psychiatrist and the neurologist and was able to secure two more prescriptions without hesitation. I presented these prescriptions to the president. He accepted them, and I was off to find the perfect dog.

We have always had dogs and I know that my husband missed having one. But it was a task to say the least. Though the dog was to be a companion for my husband, I knew that I would have to get one that was small enough for condo life and quiet enough for my pet-less community.

I began a search on the computer and John and I were both elated that we could get a dog, however small and quiet. My search began with small and friendly and very quiet dogs. Not a hyper dog – which might be yappy – but a small dog that loved to sit in someone's lap.

And there she was. A two-pound Cavachon. Such a cutie! Three months old. The cutest thing this side of the Pacific. I called the breeder and asked what kind of dog a Cavachon was. Well I learned that this teenie thing was a cross between a Cavalier King Charles and a Bichon Frise. I knew that a Bichon is a very friendly dog and loved children, but what about the King Charles? I learned that breed was very quiet and unassuming. An added plus was that the dog would not shed.

Here we are in Florida, and this little companion was in Texas. We arranged to have her shipped to us via Air transportation. It was February of 2011 when we went to Tampa International Airport to pick her up. John was so excited to see his new best friend. Now that I was able to get him a service dog to keep him company, he would not feel so alone when I had to leave.

We waited at the airport nearly an hour before we got to see our baby – who at three months, weighed two pounds. Once we got her, it was love at first sight. Now, John would be able to enjoy his new friend. But I needed to take care of some of the smaller things in his life that needed attention.

She was extremely small, but full of vinegar. Of course, she was so frightened. John was the first to hold her after removing her from her crate. And she just clung to him like a bee clings to honey. We got home and she was able to walk around and stretch her legs a bit. The next day we would begin her training.

She reminded us of a Papillion, from her coloring of white and brown to her stand-up ears. What to call her? John was cuddling her when we figured she would be called Cuddles. Perfect name for a dog that loved cuddling. The trainer came to our house to help us with her training. The trainer explained that because the puppy was so young, she would get used to people walking by our window and we would have no problem with barking. Well, this turned out to be true. She seldom barks. She is a whiner though, but fortunately it is only us that hears her. But if an egret or a heron decides to sit on our patio – beware! She does not like them nor does she appreciate the invasion of privacy! Living on the water can be interesting, to say the least. She doesn't mind the dolphins, but then again they don't have wings.

The trainer was wonderful. He told John to keep her close to his heart and she will feel his heartbeat and slow his to a normal pace as opposed to that racing or palpitating feelings he would have. I wouldn't have believed it, but it worked! Cuddles was and is a wonderful best friend for John – and also for me. Of course, she now weighs 7 pounds and does shed, but she is so worth every hair she has lost. I guess she favored the Cavalier who does shed as opposed to the Bichon Frise that does not. We are lucky to have her.

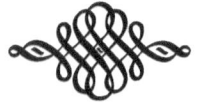

Chapter 10

Here we are a month later. Things are somewhat normal if that is what you call our life at this time.

We have been married over twenty years, and, I will add here, that they have been the best years of our lives. Of course, each of us being widowed and having children by our deceased spouses does not mean we were not happy at any other time of our lives. But reality brings us to a different era; we are now empty nesters, in a different place. Our sorrow that we share – and only we can understand – brings us together to share and develop a long-term relationship for the remainder of our lives. Only God could have created this connection. So we are, my friends, blessed. Together, we have no regrets.

Have our lives changed? Oh so much — the question is when, how, and why. We were young when we married, so we thought. At least 45 felt young, and my wonderful husband was only 55. We had so many wonderful times, and such awesome memories. Thank goodness for our memories, or should I say my memories. I will have to reminisce with my husband so that he can try to remember what fun we used to have. I have to remind myself that with Alzheimer's, I have to remember for both of us.

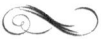

Here we go again. John was out picking up the grandchildren from school and got lost. This was a routine he did five days a week along the same roads, and he gets lost. Just think what *he* must have felt. Imagine that you are driving down a street which you drive on regularly and suddenly it becomes strange and different to you. "Where am I? Where did I turn wrong?"

"I don't recognize anything within my vision. I am scared. Oh, my God. I am lost! How did this happen? What did I do? Where did I go? Where am I going?" How frightened he must have become.

Something triggered in his brain and he forgot where he was or where he was going. Why does this happen? He was unable to recognize the sights he was once familiar with. Things he saw on a regular basis, now gone from his memory. Can we imagine the fear he must have felt? Can we understand that fear?

The school had called our son to tell him no one picked up the children, so my son immediately picked up his children and called John on his cell phone. John answered the phone and was crying and told our son he didn't know where he was.

Our son asked him what was around him and after John pointed out some landmarks, our son told him to stay there and he would drive there so that John could follow him home. When my workday was over, my son called me and asked me come to his house. I did, and John had already forgotten that he had been lost. He actually told me he was surprised to see me, as he had just dropped off the grandchildren at their home. Strange, huh? He followed me in his truck to our home.

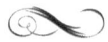

The same concern lingers daily for me. Every day, John gets up from his sleep in the morning and sits in his recliner chair and says he is miserable. He feels awful. What can I do?

We are senior citizens, but are pretty self-sufficient and can continue to live without supervision. I am the caretaker of both of us. I, for one, am still in control of my life and can take control of my beloved husband. I want him with me for a long, long time to come. We still pray each night for a long and happy life. Despite everything, I consider our life is good. But the problems are definitely building.

Lovingly, my husband is still trying to do the laundry, but I have asked him to stop putting the clothes away and to leave them folded on the bed for me to put away. It has been way too difficult for me to find the new homes my clothes have found.

I am still looking for my underwear and cannot find where he could have put it. It is like the kitchenware. If he happens to wash the dishes and pans, I have to hunt for their new locations. I try so hard to hold back my frustration – which is very nearly impossible – but I did finally find my personal items and lingerie. They had found new homes in the linen closet or in desk drawers. I decided that I now will take on another chore: from now on, I will do the laundry.

The regular routine of doing the laundry on its scheduled day has ceased, and that it's being done whenever I find time. It is more and more difficult to remember to do the laundry on a schedule, much less dry it and fold it and put it away. But at least I can put things in their proper places.

John does the dishes from time to time; it took me a week to find where he had put my pots and pans. You ought to try it. Find different places to hide things. Things that normally have a place are no longer going to be in that place and will have a brand new place all of their own.

I had to laugh, but it, of course, was frustrating. I noticed though that I had to redo the dishes before we could eat from them. Poor John couldn't see the grease or the food residue left on the plates. Add the dishes to my list of full time jobs. I already did all the cooking and now adding the dishes as well. No problem. We are still fine.

Another symptom of Alzheimer's is the clarity of sight. John told me his pain between his eyes was disturbing him constantly. He would sit in his easy chair and play solitaire on the computer day in and day out. No more driving, as he had given up his license voluntarily after getting lost. His memory of getting lost had come back to him. This was a difficult decision for him but it was a good one. The problem with giving up driving was that it takes away your independence and that can present an even bigger discouragement.

As he plays his game he rubs his eyes, John tells me he needs to have his eyes checked, as he is not seeing clearly. He has already broken a couple pair of glasses this year trying to make them sit comfortably on his nose. You know – the space where he constantly picks his face at the bridge of his nose. The nose frame irritates him due to the problems between his eyes. His constant rubbing at the top of the bridge has caused raw skin. I apply a band-aid in hopes that it will heal. Unfortunately he consistently rubs it, which will not allow the healing process. It always bleeds and has scabs. Just part of the new normal.

The aspirin and the Coumadin – both blood thinners – make his skin on his arms and hands a deep purple which irritates him. He constantly rubs these purple marks over and over with anything he can find. He will grab a fork, a knife, tweezers, scissors, cuticle clippers, even a toothpick. I am told all this picking is a part of the disease. But why does this happen? He is making his skin twice as bad. So a disease that causes memory loss also is the perpetrator of several other types of eccentricities?

Well he wants to get an eye exam. He had one six months ago but is now complaining that his eyeglasses are not clear and he is having trouble seeing. I explain that the computer screen can cause problems when one stares at it constantly. Maybe he should rest his eyes every so often from playing the computer and go back to it later.

Well, that works for five minutes, as he has forgotten that he isn't seeing so well. This, too, is a result of Alzheimer's. The vision suffers from blurriness and lack of clarity. This probably causes those with glasses to complain that their glasses are old and that they need a new prescription. I'll experience more of this later, as I came to find out.

A couple of weeks went by and, again, John and I are talking about his problems, one of which is his eyeglasses. He tells me he cannot see very well out of his glasses. Since the last eye exam was such a short time ago – less than a year – he wants me to make an appointment for a new eye exam. I find an old pair of glasses that are probably two or more years old and give them to him to see if he likes those better and, low and behold, he does!

He wears them for about three or four hours, but then complains again, so I exchange them for the newest ones he has. Now he likes those again, so he will wear those until the next time he complains. No doubt that will be in a few weeks.

Today is another frustrating day. I am nearly afraid to ask my loving husband how he is. His answer is always the same: lousy. I feel lousy. "What can I do to help? What is the problem? Can I do something to make you feel better?" I ask. All my questions go unanswered. Such a terrible time we are having in our lives. John sits in his chair and looks hopeless. He sits there day after day in his pajamas, same clothes from the day before, no shower without my pleading. Getting him to change into street clothes is next to impossible. He complains, asking why he should when we aren't going anywhere anyway. What do I do to convince him that he will feel better if he changes clothes, even if he is only pretending that he has somewhere to go? This is draining for me. Where do I go from here?

It tires me out, this pleading, the begging him to shower, the convincing him to dress. It becomes more and more clear, as I'm sure it does to you, dear reader, that I need help. My physical exhaustion is obvious, and my mental exhaustion is definitely taking a toll. I do not want my precious husband to see me cry, because I do not have any regrets and I won't allow him to blame himself or feel that he is a burden to me. I do not regret anything other than I am losing him to this unspeakable disease.

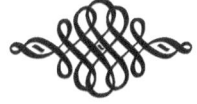

Chapter 11

It happened again. John took my medication without my knowledge, except that this time he realized that he did take it and was concerned about his reaction to it.

I called 911 and told them of his previous reaction to my meds and they advised that I bring him to the hospital for admission. He spent two days under observation, and was released. He turned out fine. Actually he did better this time than he did the first time he took my meds.

But the hospital took its toll on him. He was so uncomfortable not knowing or understanding where he was confined. When he at last came home, he relaxed in the familiar environment. Another sign of Alzheimer's is the confusion and anxiety they feel when leaving their familiar place. John has this textbook symptom.

Weeks come to an end and new weeks begin, but change, though gradual and deliberate, wears and wears.

Eventually, this crippling disease will capture the entire mind of our loved one.

Life as I have known it over the past twenty years will never be the same. I can handle it, but I still have questions. I ask the doctors, please tell me why is my husband in pain at his forehead? I was not aware that dementia caused pain.

John described the pain as more like discomfort, "like a fluttering in my forehead, and it is just so annoying," he said. I asked him if it hurt like a headache, and he said no, but that it was so disturbing it kept him from concentrating.

I ask the doctors, what is this problem? Can we make this irritation go away? Can we help my husband? In order to not complain, my husband tells the doctor he is not in pain but just uncomfortable. I am sure this will change back to "pain" soon enough.

I continue my struggle to find relief for my husband, so that this disease which is making its home within my husbands head can be put to sleep. Oddly, I wish that forgetfulness was the only nasty symptom we had to deal with.

The doctors have said they are sorry, but the nature of the disease is different for everyone. The discomfort my husband feels cannot be diagnosed. CAT scans, MRI's, X-rays, you name it, all have been done and the results have shown nothing wrong. But he feels *something*, and though I am not a part of it, I feel something too. It is not pain I feel, but frustration for his discomfort.

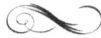

Next stop: a psychiatrist. We are still in 2010, and it is an important year as things begin to speed up. We again visit our neurologist, who in turn recommends we see a psychiatrist. We call him and set an appointment to speak with him. Perhaps, it is a last ditch effort. Perhaps, he will help.

So far, the doctors we have seen are not for his memory or that he has the start of Alzheimer's, but for the discomfort he feels. Yes, I know what dementia is and I saw it first-hand with my mother and now I see it with my husband. It does not shock me; I am aware of its debilitating process.

I don't want to deal with this, but I am trying hard not to ignore it or disbelieve it. You know – that denial stage. I am not denying it, but trying so hard to *fight* it. Maybe, I can fix it; maybe, I can put it on the back burner. I tell the disease to come back in a few years, to let us have a few more sane years left in our marriage before it takes my husband away. This is not right. But, then again, what is fair? We have so much more we have to do and see and feel. Please, we don't have time for this. We could have so many more good years. Let me keep trying to salvage what we have left.

Onward and upward. We visited the psychiatrist. He asked us many questions about what was happening. We told the doctor about one of the key issues we are having: lack of energy. John says he does not have the energy to take a shower or get dressed or to participate in life. He can't even concentrate on television. Watching television was not a pleasure anymore, but a chore. The commercials interfered with his memory of the show. For someone with this disease, watching television is difficult to follow due to the interruptions of each scene with commercials and editing. The frequent changes create the inability to follow for someone lacking in memory skills.

The doctor even asked John, "Do you ever feel like hurting yourself?"

"Not at all," my husband explained, adding, "Though my memory is so bad I often feel sad that I am losing it."

Remember, people with this disease know what is happening to them. This is devastating to them, and they want to either deny it or work through it, somehow hiding it or rising above it to fight it. They themselves – and their caregivers – study the symptoms to see what they can do to slow down the process. Can foods slow the process? Can medications or reading more or doing puzzles slow it down? How about never quitting work? If one just doesn't retire, will it slow down the spread of the disease? Is this what is in store for us as we age gracefully? Do we continue to work till we die so that we can die with dignity? Or do we retire to enjoy the twilight of our lives, only to find ourselves being sedate and stagnant inviting the disease to enter our lives to fill the emptiness we now feel? Answers are hard to come by.

Our independence is slipping away. Our youthfulness deteriorates, leaving us older folks – if we're lucky – with memories of times gone by. And, if we're not lucky, with a disease that takes our treasured moments from us.

This new doctor explained to us that a lot of the problems that John faced was due to the depression that seeps in as the forgetfulness progresses. We know what is happening, yet we cannot control it. John remembers when he sees his children, but shortly after their departure he forgets they had visited. Then he becomes sad when he realizes he forgot. He becomes angry when he realizes he cannot control his memory.

"It's blank inside. I have no memory at all of the event," he tells me. "When were they here? How long did they stay? What is happening in their lives? Am I forgetting something important?"

I have no answers for him.

The other day, I asked him to name the months that his three sons were born in. I, myself, can remember the months but still struggle with the particular day. Again, sadness overcomes him because he can't even remember the days or the months in which his children were born.

So far, I feel content that he has remembered our twenty years together. I am blessed, indeed. I hope that the memories we share do not fade. I will continue to reminisce. I will keep the memories alive and up front within reach of just a thought.

After much discussion, the doctor suggested that we check out some new medications to at least help with John's severe depression.

The psychiatrist suggested that John be hospitalized in a local sanitarium for one week while they try to find what medications or combination of medicines will help with the sadness and the weeping. So, John entered a local sanitarium, where all patients are in lockdown. No one was allowed to visit except at posted visitation hours – only two hours a day between 6PM and 8PM. I had to drop him off at the hospital and was told I could leave and come back later. With a heavy heart, I dropped him off.

I returned as soon as I could. I was amazed and shocked to find my husband wearing his same clothes, but missing his belt, and his shoes replaced by hospital socks. See, I had left clothes for him to change into, but he was not able to remember and no one was there to remind him. This was a sanitarium, not a hospital, and the level of care was much different. A hospital is more hands-on; here he is left on his own, observed, and given medication to gauge its effectiveness.

A couple of days went by, and he was beginning to get that scruffy-beard look. The next day, I brought him his electric shaver, but they confiscated it because of the cord, and they would never remind him to shave anyway. Of course, John couldn't remember to shave, either.

I was a bit miffed to find his beard getting heavier. The nursing staff explained to me that the cord presents a danger not only to himself, but to others in the ward that could steal it. I really hated him being there; the level of care was less than I had expected. And, of course, because it was a private sanitarium, the cost was not covered by Medicare or the supplemental insurance company. It was costing in excess of $300.00 per day.

It was a lock-down unit, and I knew he would be safe. Whatever the experience was, it was to help him and that would be what I needed to keep in mind.

When I visited him, I struggled with his believing that this was his new home. He even told me he liked it there. I was sad and tried to convince him this was only for one week, but it was so difficult for him to remember or understand. I was upset that he felt I had made him move there without me. We had planned a trip for his birthday, which was fast approaching, and I was hoping that once he got home he would remember his surroundings. He stayed at the facility, with the time for the trip ticking down.

At last, the day came when the doctor was ready to release John, one day later than planned. He was released the very day that we were to leave for Orlando for the vacation.

On our way home John asked me why I took him out of his "new home," the sanitarium. This nearly broke my heart. I reminded him he was only there for one week (well, eight days) to regulate his medication. I brought him back to our home so that he could shave and shower and put on some clean clothes. I would pack up the car for our trip.

It was difficult for me while he was in the facility. A lockdown building that I could visit but not be allowed to walk in without signing in or wearing a visitors tag – not the homiest of places. I am sure it was to protect the other patients who wanted to leave without permission. There were all types of patients there, from teens on drugs to seniors not wanting to live.

I noticed that just putting him in this facility was enough to add to his considerable disorientation. Afterwards, I told the doctor about the lack of care John received. The doctor explained, that considering that

John has dementia, it was much better for him to be in a unit with people much like himself – quiet, unpretentious, inconspicuous – than it would be in a psychiatric unit at a hospital where all people are in the same unit regardless of the level of care they needed. Anger issues, alcohol abuse, drug abuse and dementia, all on the same floor in the same section. I suppose the doctor was right; any of that arrogant, nasty, or outrageous behavior would not have set well with my husband.

I worried about my husband coming home two hours before we were to leave for our family reunion. He cried – or should I say sobbed – on the way home, asking me why I took him out of his home. I was shocked and saddened by this revelation. What have I done? Is this confusion due to something I did in my search to hold on to him? Good Lord, what have I done?

When we arrived home, things came back to him – a bit. He seemed to recognize the familiar surroundings. Sitting in his easy chair and hugging his little dog, Cuddles, he seemed to be happier. He began to come around, but we were in a hurry.

First thing was for him to shave. While I was making him lunch and packed the car, I gave him his razor. He shaved, took a supervised shower and dressed. In a hurry, we hit the road.

We picked up our three grandchildren from school and drove to our destination. The other family members would be there a few hours after us. We were quite content. John seemed to have it together. All seemed to be going just fine, and the trip was uneventful.

The family all arrived in the early evening. We had a fun night checking out our rooms, which were gorgeous. We had five bedrooms and four bathrooms. Our master bedroom had a beautiful bath in it. After visiting with each other we all went to bed. John and I went to our master bedroom and fell totally asleep ... or so I thought.

I had assumed that it would be an uneventful night. Well, you know what they say about assuming anything. True to form, my night was truly about to begin.

Through my sleep, I thought I heard a noise. I rolled over, and John wasn't in bed. I called out to him, but heard nothing. *He must be in the bathroom*, I thought. I called out again, and, again, silence. I got up to check.

He was not in our master bathroom, so I opened the door and called out to him to see if he was in the second bathroom, but again to no avail. I ended up waking Paul, my stepson, during my search. Paul asked me what was going on. I told him I couldn't find his dad. So then the normal questions came up: is he in the bathroom, etc... Cuddles, the little companion dog, was soundly sleeping in the bed, but John was nowhere to be found. We searched the entire apartment, but no sign of John.

As a last effort, we went to the front door, which was the typical hotel type that locks behind you when you exit the room. John would never exit the room though, would he? I peeked outside.

"Oh dear, Paul, there he is lying on the floor at the end of the hallway!" I exclaimed.

It was 3:15 in the morning and there was my sweet husband on the floor in the hallway about 8 or 9 doors down. *Oh God, I hope he is just asleep*, I thought. Paul ran down to him , and I ran in to get the wheelchair. John was fine, but in his search for a bathroom, being disoriented, he lost focus as to where he was. Poor John was so confused he totally lost his whereabouts and left the room in his jockey shorts. We brought him back to the unit, he got to go to the bathroom, and finally we all got back to sleep.

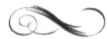

All was well for the next few days. We made provisions to prevent a repeat of the first night. We put a large chair in front of the door that would totally encumber his move out the door again. If John was going to try and leave the unit again, we would hear him.

I truly believe that the stay at the sanitarium confused his thinking. The change caused John disorientation and had taken him out of his comfort zone. This is a symptom of the illness, one not as well known, but still an important one. That is why so often my husband would refuse to leave the comfort of his home where he felt safe.

We had a wonderful reunion for the remainder of the time. Again, there was the sadness as our families departed for their northern destinations. But it was good to spend time with them, however passing it was.

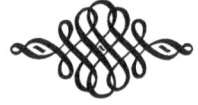

Chapter 12

Here it is, 2011, and time is fleeting by almost as fast as John's memory. His medications now include Namenda and Razadyne both memory enhancers, plus three different anti-depressants.

Now, you may ask, are the memory medications working? I don't really know. I questioned this as well as you might be. I even asked the doctors that very question. The answer I received was this: only you would know. Well, it was hard to tell.

The medication does not stop the process but only slows it down. The diagnosis is there, and the prognosis is this disease will take his life at some point. What kind of a gamble is this? You can always stop the medication and see what happens or continue on hoping that the process has slowed down. But how do I know? The answer is that it is a major gamble. Would you be willing to take it?

What a scary choice – to see if the medications are working by stopping them, then, if he deteriorates faster, to reintroduce them but have him be at a new, poorer condition. Do I really want to take on that type of gamble?

Of course, it is a lose-lose situation; there will be no gamble with my husband's memory. We will continue the medications until we are sure they will no longer help. These particular medications are also among the most expensive on the market. This horrendous disease is not only terminal, but long-term terminal – not a shortened, quick peril but a long, unrelenting sickness that strips the life and dignity of the human mind.

Let me explain the new place where we are now. We are on a roll at the top of Alzheimer's, and this is a rolling ball that is picking up speed and ready to flatten us. At home, we no longer have conversations. Watching television together has become of thing of the past. I wondered why he no longer was interested in his beloved football. What happened to the baseball games? Why? The brain is very complex and the part of the brain called the amygdala – the part containing the memories – is now deteriorating. With the memories gone, it does not just affect the things we reminisce about or what you ate or where you went. The disease is so much more heartless than that.

John can no longer concentrate or think or keep up with conversation. My husband and I would drink a glass or two of wine in the evening. But usually it was when our dog was in his lap and he was playing solitaire. How was he able to play solitaire? This is beyond my wildest imagination. How is he still able to know what he is doing? But this brings a smile to my face. His ability to wile away the day is awesome, for now. The brain activity, we are told, can continue to function normally until the complete breakdown of the amygdala.

Of course, he doesn't remember to take the dog out for relief, or feed himself, or even make sure our dog has fresh water. We still go for Coumadin checks and to see physicians as needed. The picking of his skin is still a major concern. He still knows my name, but does struggle with those he does not see on a daily basis – the children or the grandchildren.

Life continues to pass by, taking us along. I struggle with having John go out to appointments. I also struggle going out myself and leaving him alone, which he really hates as he fears dying alone.

I noticed that his eating habits have changed dramatically. He does not recognize steak from chicken from hamburger. He asks me if he likes it. Normally, he eats with two hands, but now I see him eating with only one hand almost as if his right hand hurts to move. He enjoys breakfast and supper, but not lunch. I still struggle with his hygiene, but after speaking to the doctor about it, I will be getting some help within a couple of months. The New Year is coming, maybe it will bring with it new solutions and changes for the better.

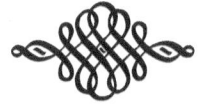

Chapter 13

It's March of 2012, and I really want to go on a cruise. It has been several years since we have gone. I ask my sweetheart if he wanted to go on a cruise and – lo and behold – his answer was a vibrant "yes!" Oh, my God, let me set this up before he changes his mind! I know he will forget, but I will remind him daily about the cruise. Then it dawns on me – it will probably be my last vacation with him. So, I hurry and book the cruise for late August of 2012. He is in a wheelchair now, and all I have to do is push him around the ship. Of course, as a service dog, Cuddles also gets to go, which will please John.

With the cruise in place, we go on with the rest of the stuff going on in our lives. We have company come to visit us for a few days. I tell John who they are and he does not remember them, at least not by name. But hopefully when he sees them, he will recognize their faces. They arrive, and John says he remembers them, but again I know he is trying to remember but really cannot. This makes him uneasy, but he understands that we obviously know them. Our friends and I make conversation, but John sits and plays with Cuddles.

Our friends mention that they want to go bowling. They want to see our entire family, so why not have us all meet at the bowling alley and really have some fun? So off we go, the entire family – including grandchildren and children. The only one that didn't get to come was Cuddles.

John sat in his wheelchair and was going to watch. I can't explain what happened next or what triggered it, but it was certainly dramatic.

Everyone put on the bowling shoes and left their sneakers on the floor near the wheelchair. The noise factor in the bowling alley must have hit 150 decibels. John was physically at the alley, but mentally had withdrawn into himself. He picked up a sneaker and unlaced it, re-laced it, and unlaced it. Then, he acted like he was going to drink from it! I went over to him to see if he wanted something, but to my dismay he could not see me. I tried to have him look at me, but he could not focus for some reason. He didn't see me, but looked through me as if I were not there. I thought maybe he was thirsty, so I bought him a hot dog and a cold drink. He obviously was hungry because he voraciously ate the hotdog. I turned a moment, and my children grabbed me right away; he was also eating the wrapper. I pulled the paper from his mouth and he was fine. I gave him his cold soda and he drank.

Now my children were panic-stricken and begging me not to go on the cruise I had planned for August with John, as it would leave me rattled to say the least. My daughter was going on the cruise with me and became extremely concerned about her stepdad's wellbeing. She also wanted me to cancel the trip, but I really felt that the ship had to be a lot quieter, as opposed to the noise of the bowling alley.

We finished our game and went home where all was well. The only concern John had was who were the people staying with us. Didn't they have their own place? I again explained they were our guests and were here for just a few days to visit us.

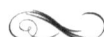

In the peace and quiet of home, all appears to be fine. John plays with his dog and takes a break from his computer game and just sits with me. We have some potato chips and enjoy a glass of wine. Then, I notice something new happening to my honey.

He wants another glass of wine. "Okay dear, hand me your wine glass". Hey, is wine good without a stemmed wine glass? Not for us anyway. John asks where his glass is. I tell him it is right on his side table, with the chips he was eating. He hands me the box of tissues. What? The wine glass, John. Oh, he says, and hands me the bag of chips. Is he playing with me? What is going on? "Honey the glass you just drank the wine from," I tell him.

The glass is on the table next to the phone. He studies the table, but does not see it. What happened? This is very strange to me. I decide not to ask again and I get up and pick up his glass and pour some wine into it.

John says, "Oh that's what you wanted, why didn't you say so."

I sit back down and just watch television while my head spins and spins.

One day, I called him while I was running errands. I knew he would be hungry, so I told him to go in the kitchen and take the sandwich I had made from the fridge. He told me he didn't know where the fridge was. We all have portable phones so I told him to walk to the kitchen and I would walk him through the steps to find the sandwich. This is what it is like living with Alzheimer's:

John is in the kitchen.

Open the refrigerator and look in, I tell him.

"Okay, I don't see anything like a sandwich."

"It's on the bottom shelf, right next to the orange juice."

He says he can't find the orange juice. Then he says he will wait until I get home. His frustration was making him anxious. I didn't push it any further. I had placed the sandwich on the bottom shelf of the refrigerator at the front between the milk and the orange juice, trying to make it obvious.

Was this a problem he was having with his eyeglasses? Are they blurring his vision enough that he cannot see things? I made an appointment for us both to get our eyes tested. Maybe he was right, the glasses were the wrong prescription, or this disease has affected his eyes and he needs to have them checked again.

I did learn later that Alzheimer's does affect the eyes and the way victims see. The vision becomes blurred and makes the patient unable to focus. What a horrendous disease. Everyday, this evil perpetrator reveals a new symptom.

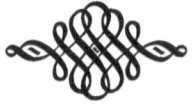

Chapter 14

The time for our cruise is fast approaching. I tell John we should empty out our five-gallon water jug of all the change we have been saving through these past few years. We will be able to have this extra money for our cruise. So I set up the card table and cover it with a large white towel to pour out the change so that it doesn't bounce on the floor. John picks up a couple of coins and stares at them as if he has never seen one before. I really don't pay that much attention, as he used to collect coins and research them looking for that million dollar coin. I ask him to help me by separating the pennies, dimes, nickels and quarters.

This is new to him. He looks over the pennies and dimes and places them in one pile. Then asks me what the nickels were. He was unable to place them apart from the quarters. I carefully watched him as I continued to separate the coins. I could see the frustration on his face, his difficulty in deciding which were pennies and which were dimes. My heart broke. He has forgotten the coins and their denominations as well as their worth. I watched as his anxiety flushed through his body; he began to cry and become angry at himself, and this disease. I told him it was okay, that I would take care of the coins. I wrapped and deposited in our account a few days later.

Here we are the morning of our cruise. We are all packed and ready to go. We have to go to Port Canaveral, which is about three hours away by car. All is well. There are four of us, plus our dog, and we are all excited, even John.

I knew this would be good for us because we have been on fourteen cruises up to this one, so he should be able to find some memory of them. Each cruise was better than the last – we so enjoy them.

This time, John would be in a wheel chair which will help him with his walking since he really can't walk long distances. He falls so much I finally bought a bed rail to keep him in bed and my back in one piece since he weighs so much. He was able to walk short distances back and forth at home as he went to the bedroom or to the bathroom, but these ships are huge and there's a lot of walking. The wheelchair was a necessity.

Between the three of us, we would be able to push the wheelchair anywhere we wanted to go and taking turns would be greatly helpful. The ship is certainly equipped to accept handicapped people with the bathrooms so handy, though I found the archways between the cabins a bit high and difficult to negotiate with a heavy wheelchair. But, in general, people are kind – if I was struggling, there would always be someone to lend assistance.

Getting to Port Canaveral was fairly uneventful. I can honestly say my expectations were a lot less comfortable than how we actually fared. The only question during the ride was "Are we there yet"?

Boarding the ship was smooth, probably due to our Royal Crown Membership. This was a fabulous day. We went to our respective cabins to check them out and drop off the items we had carried onto the ship.

We decided to eat as we were all pretty hungry, so we went up to the Windjammer Cafeteria which is the same on all Royal Caribbean Ships. We had a great lunch. John was on cloud nine, and my daughter and I were so happy we were bursting with joy at John's total reaction to the ship. He remembers bits and pieces – this is awesome.

Cuddles, our little seven-pound Cavachon, was the delight of the ship. Each person we passed stopped to talk and John was so happy to talk about his baby. He was able to remember the dog's name but that was about it. The afternoon went along these lines: "Hi, what a cute dog!" or "Oh, wow, look at that cute dog!" and ,"Oh my goodness, what kind of a dog is that?" It was a good day.

We wandered about this massive ship, which held about five thousand people. Throughout the seven-day cruise, I believe John said "hi" to more than half of the passengers who stopped to pet Cuddles. We were the only family aboard that had brought our service animal with us, and with her weight at a slight seven pounds, she certainly created a warm stir and a large welcome.

We went down for supper, and the ship was on its way. The meal was decadent. We enjoyed wine with our meal while our baby just slept under the table for a much needed rest.

As the days flew by only a few situations cropped up. One evening, on retiring from the day's activities, we fell asleep quickly. At about six AM, I was awakened by my husband. I asked if he was alright.

"Of course, but I have to get ready for work," he replied.

Uh oh.

I reminded him that he was retired.

"I know, but I don't want to be late for work," he insisted.

I knew this was going to take some convincing. I accomplished getting him back into bed by telling him it was okay to miss this day because I already called in to report him sick.

"Oh that's good, so I guess it won't hurt to miss a day," he reasoned.

I agreed, and John came back to bed. Perhaps he had been in a deep dream, remembering the past. Perhaps the Alzheimer's had crossed his cables. Who knows?

Another day, he asked why our new house was so small – meaning the cabin. I reminded him that we were in a small cabin on a cruise ship. He became comfortable again. At least that one was an easy one.

The most important problem that arose was John's bathroom ablutions. A new duty had arisen for me. We were back at our cabin, where John had to use the facility. He was in there so long, I interrupted him. I opened the door to see what he was doing. He was just sitting there, confused and embarrassed; he told me he was trying to figure out how he would clean himself. I was so sad for him. How awful for him to lose this dignity along with all the other things he was losing. At least I was grateful that he realized that he needed cleaning. I understand that somewhere further into the illness all bathroom habits are lost. Lucky me, my husband was a very proud man and still in control of his elimination ability, just a little help from his beloved wife will be all he needs. I took on my new responsibility without hesitation. Whatever my husband needs, I am at his side. For better or worse were part of our vows, and now my husband needs me more than ever. I am proud to do what I can to help my sweetheart in his time of need. From this point forward, I accompanied my husband to the handicapped restrooms on the ship.

We enjoyed our daily stroll through the promenade on the "Freedom of the Seas". We found tea and coffee shops where we could stop for a snack while my daughter enjoyed her cruise. We had already been to each of the ports, so not leaving the ship was fine for us.

Sometimes when I was pushing and looking at my sweet husband, I could see that some quiet time was needed. While my daughter and her friend disembarked from the ship to take in the sights, John and I would find a quiet lounge where we could have a glass of wine and I could read my book and he would relax playing his solitaire.

Of course, not everyone left the ship. A few folks like us stayed aboard and enjoyed the amenities. While I was reading my book, John asked me why all these strange people were walking through our home. Oh, I knew he had once again forgotten that we were on a cruise; just a reminder settled him down.

The second to the last night was a formal night. I knew it was time to go home; John had had enough. I tried to help him get dressed, but he was not having it. I could feel his anxiety and did not push the change of clothes. I told him we could go to dinner as he was, and Cuddles will also go along. This definitely calmed him down.

How did our dog calm him down, you ask? It was amazing. John would hold her close and she would kiss him and lay her head on his chest and he would stop thinking about his anxious feelings and just give her love and receive love in return. Evidently, love is all it takes. Love that is physical and endearing. Love from man's best friend. An animal can supply the love and security that one may need – that unconditional love that only a pet can give. The love they give regardless of the situation. Whether you are sitting, struggling, angry or lethargic, a pet will love you and always be with you. The best medicine I ever got for my husband was that beloved dog. This medicine doesn't have to be refilled, has no uncomfortable side effects and doesn't talk back, but will listen intently.

So, back to the formal night. I had struggled daily dressing him since we boarded. I was fairly used to that. We proceeded to the dining room with the three of us dressed in our best, and John still in his Bermuda shorts.

In the dining area, people everywhere were in long dresses and suits. John got a bit miffed at me for not telling him it was a formal night. I tried not to roll my eyes. I asked him if he was comfortable and he told me he was, I in turn said fine, you look great. As Hospice would tell me, you pick your arguments, and that one just seemed like it did not need to be thrashed out.

Early on, I remember becoming frustrated with the disease and all the questions he didn't understand. So many times I, as the caregiver, would feel anger when he was unable to answer questions that I would ask. In the beginning, I drove everywhere we needed to go and he would say are we going the wrong way, as this does not look familiar. Now, it doesn't faze me – much.

We are husband and wife and we talk, but remembering for John is a thing of the past. Remembering for me has doubled, though, because as life flies by, I have to remember that John does *not* remember, and that can be exasperating. It's not a daily ritual to see things that are happening to him, but on occasion – and that is saying when we disagree – it is up to me to remember his condition. Once I was able to get my head around the disease, I saw what would bring on the anxiety attacks. Everything in our lives must be quiet and relaxed; this will keep him calm.

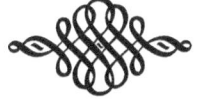

Chapter 15

The cruise is over, and we had a great time. I am so glad we went. John says he had a great time, too. I know Cuddles made about three thousand friends, and that was wonderful. We are now homeward bound to our ordinary lives.

We're back at home now, where things seem to be speeding up. It's as if this disease takes on a life of its own and has now become a roller coaster. At night, my husband asks me where I want him to sleep. Upstairs or down stairs, yet we live in a one-story villa. Sometimes, I think he is seeing things. He asks who the people are in our house when we are completely alone.

Maybe his mind is still on the ship where there were people all around us walking. I don't really know where his mind is. Our home is quiet and we are sedentary. I am not sure where he is in his brain.

What is happening? This memory loss is creating other strange things, with hallucinating now a new tentacle of this atrocious disease. I stare into space myself, begging to understand. John is not playing his computer solitaire game. I see him pick it up and play solitaire for a couple of hours, but by no means is he playing for the normal eight hours a day. I see him play with the dog, stare out the window at the water, or stare into space.

I remind him to play and he tells me he does not feel like it. A few times I open the computer to his game and place it on his lap so that he can play the game as he was accustomed to doing. The computer seems to have slipped from his daily routine. When I put the computer on his lap I see him look at it in dismay and then close it up. I ask why and his answer is he is tired of it, but I know he can't remember how. My poor husband – this cruel disease has taken the spirit for living out of his life. No television, no computer to while away the hours while he is just sitting.

It's Fall, and we in Florida do not have leaves changing, so the only view is the water of Tampa Bay. I am at least happy that it is such a beautiful view. To watch the "big fish," as John calls the dolphin, or to watch a boat scoot by with eager fishermen or the jet skis is so much fun.

But to watch him as he just looks into space is just destroying me. At least we now have hospice support system helping him with his showers. This makes him feel like he has company, and he enjoys it. I also enjoy them as they come by to visit and hear about his progress or, better said, his regress. They are one of the best support systems ever to have graced this earth.

It is now October 7, 2012 and we are watching television and relaxing. My sweetheart has to go to the bathroom, so I help him go and tell him to call me when he needs me. I hear him calling me so I go to him and he is on the floor in the bedroom – he had walked out of the bathroom by himself and slipped and fell. I asked him if he was okay and he said he was, so I asked him to use the night table to help himself get up.

He was confused as to what I was saying. "Honey get on your knees," I tell him, and he looks at me as if I were speaking a foreign language. I tried to bend his legs to help him kneel, to no avail.

He weighs 280 pounds and on the floor he is dead weight. No way I can pick him up. This is an impossible task for me.

"John, honey, sit there while I call 911," I tell him.

I do, and ask for lift assistance. The fire department was here in no time. Unfortunately, the two skinny guys took one look at John and sent for more power and strength. Another fellow came and together they helped him up. I asked them to please put him in his easy chair and they told me they would check his vitals. A fireman told me John had a fever. I didn't know that, they advised me it was best to take John to the hospital to have him checked out. It was a low-grade fever, but better to check him and be sure.

But John told me he was fine. Again, I asked them to just put him back in his easy chair. They told me they could not. I guess they have a responsibility to be sure his condition was good.

As they loaded him in the ambulance, the EMT's told me to wait a half-hour before driving to the hospital so they would have time to transfer him and take vitals.

I drove myself to the hospital and asked the woman at the desk to let me into the emergency area where my husband was. She was gracious and allowed me entry.

Once the doors opened, I could see my sweetheart in the room down the hall from where I stood.

I hurried to him, and when I leaned in to give him a kiss I noticed that his pillow was soaked through and through. His sheets were soaked, too, and sweat from his head was pouring down his face. What the hell is this? Why is he so hot? Nurses came in and checked on him. I told him he needed dry sheets and a dry pillowcase, the ones he had were absolutely saturated.

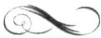

I called my son who lives nearby, and John's son who lived nearby in Palmetto. My son arrived first, and my stepson a little while later. We were all concerned about his perspiring and wanted to know why this was happening to him.

He was tested and the cause of the high fever was not found. I was beside myself; my husband came here because he fell down and I could not lift him up. Why does he have a high fever? All this is new, and in less than two hours. What is happening? I don't understand.

The attending doctor decided John would be admitted so that they could try to determine where this fever of 104 degrees came from. He told me to go home, that he was stable and would be fine tonight. They would watch him carefully, they promised. I decided he was in good hands, and I needed to go home and rest so that I would come back tomorrow refreshed.

The next day, I was preparing to return to the hospital to see how my sweetheart was doing. He was fine when he left our home, so I thought. After all, he had only fallen on the floor and I was unable to pick him up. Okay, so I didn't know he had a fever – but then again he wasn't complaining about being sick. He didn't *look* sick. He only fell on the floor. I only needed help picking him up and putting him in his easy chair.

I arrived at the hospital and John seemed awful. He was nearly delirious, and his son, David and his wife, Karen arrived and agreed that he looked dreadful and was not at all himself. It gave us quite the scare. What the hell happened overnight? My son and his wife arrived, and they too were totally disturbed by what they saw.

My stepson called his brothers to explain this latest turn of events. It didn't look good. My son and daughter came to see their step-dad, and were also upset at his poor condition. He was unable to talk and explain how he was feeling. What is going on? He fell on the floor – all he needed was help to get back on his feet. Again, I expressed, what the hell happened?

He was on all kinds of medications, with needles through his arms and under the continuous watch of nurses. The family took turns staying with him that day.

At night, we went home concerned about the condition we left John in. We all returned early the next day, and, to our great relief, John had greatly improved. He saw me and was genuinely excited to see me. Hurrah. His son and his wife arrived and were so relieved to see him alert and better.

Wow, sweetheart you scared me, I whispered to him.

A day ago, my stepson had called his brothers to explain to them that they needed to fly down to say their good byes. Today, John looks and acts so good, that another call goes through to cancel the emergency flights.

Thank goodness he appeared better. We all relaxed.

The next day we arrived to find John in a state of confusion and disoriented. What was going on? His breathing was labored and he was unable to speak and seemed to be getting worse again.

Another phone call goes out to my stepsons to reiterate what the first phone call had declared – we are in trouble here. You need to hop a plane and come here to see your dad, my stepson told them.

Wait a minute, John only fell. What the hell is going on? Who is in charge? It was time to speak to someone with authority. John's breathing was so labored. An oxygen specialist arrived and was quite disturbed that John was not in intensive care. His breathing was so labored and he was exhausted just trying to breathe. The specialist gave him a breathing treatment to ease the work of the lungs. The entire family had arrived to see the situation at hand. We were all so confused ourselves.

Things started to move. This technician was wonderful, as he was doing everything humanly possible to bring comfort to my sweetheart. After a long, long day, it was time to go home and see what the next day would bring.

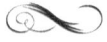

The next day, the entire family gathered. Dr. Rajani, the physician attending my husband decided to speak with all of us. After looking at the medical records, he asked me if John had a living will, which he did. The doctor asked me to bring it to the hospital and then talked to us about end of life. My mind spun; my world spun. My husband only fell. What was this doctor talking about? What had happened?

The doctor explained that John had been sick and it went undetected for a few days. When he fell, it made it possible to find it. The doctor explained that John had pneumonia and the medications they have him on are the absolute strongest ones available. The doctor explained that the Alzheimer's was preventing the medications from working normally. The brain controlled all the problems that were affecting John. They had exhausted their resources to help him, and what they had done was not working. The doctor asked if we wanted to let nature take its course. What? He only fell, I protested. Yes, but had he not fallen, he would have ended up in the hospital the next few days anyway. The illness would have presented itself eventually.

What to do? My decision weighs heavy on my heart. This is my soul mate, my lover, my companion, my best friend, my everything. The doctor tells us, my entire family, my children, John's children, their wives and our oldest grandchildren, that if John survives this – and it is possible but improbable because the medicines they are giving him intravenously are not even making a dent in his condition – John would be brought back to the hospital in another two weeks for some other problem. I am grateful that my oldest granddaughter, Tayla, is in attendance as she has just recently graduated from college where she majored in Pharmacology. We all depend on her to explain the type of drugs being administered to John. I am sincerely grateful to her for the support she offers me.

This is how Alzheimer's works I'm told – by preventing the brain from functioning normally. The doctors heal us with medicines they prescribe. We benefit from their knowledge and the care we receive. But it is our brain that must work together with the treatment plan. When the brain dies, we are nothing but a vegetable unable to control any function. This would be the state the body takes when the brain stops functioning; the state that allows donors to give working body parts to recipients who can still function in our world. I hear all this in a numb haze as I look upon my husband.

We stay in a private room and my husband fights the inevitable. Why, oh why, is this happening? I love him; I don't mind taking care of him. I have never really complained. Oh yes, I have vented, but isn't that normal in order to hold on to sanity? Do I want him to die with dignity, or does that matter? I didn't think that death was that close at hand. Okay, okay so he was deteriorating at a frightening speed, but do I want to give up? John is my world, my whole life. I am so scared. His breathing is more and more labored. My poor sweetheart is struggling to get air to his lungs. Help him, please. I can't stand to watch him struggle so. His pain is my pain.

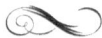

We sleep at the hospital in the private room, where we can stay with him every moment. The entire family is with him. He can hear us, I am sure, but he is unable to respond, and I am sad. I sing to him and talk to him and kiss him and I am sure he knows this. He tries to acknowledge my kiss and my love.

We are surrounded by our family feeling lots of love. I see my husband struggling for air as he tries to breathe. Lord, help him. I hurt for him. It is October 21, 2012 and he is breathing with the help of the oxygen placed on his nose.

The air is forced into his lungs. We can hear it as it enters and exits his lungs. We all talk to him and express our love. He must feel the love and warmth we give him.

The night comes and goes in a blur, and a new morning dawns. I talk to John and tell him my love is so strong that it will cure anything, but if the Lord has decided that this is the time for him to come home, then so be it. I tell my loving husband to reach out and hold the hand of Jesus, and follow the light he sees.

It is October 22, 2012, and the oxygen runs out. The nurse comes in to replace it, and I tell her to leave us alone. I kiss my husband good bye and tell him I love him. He takes that last breath and envelops me with all the love he conveys to me. I feel his spirit in the room as we all bid to my husband, a father, and a grandfather farewell on his final journey home.

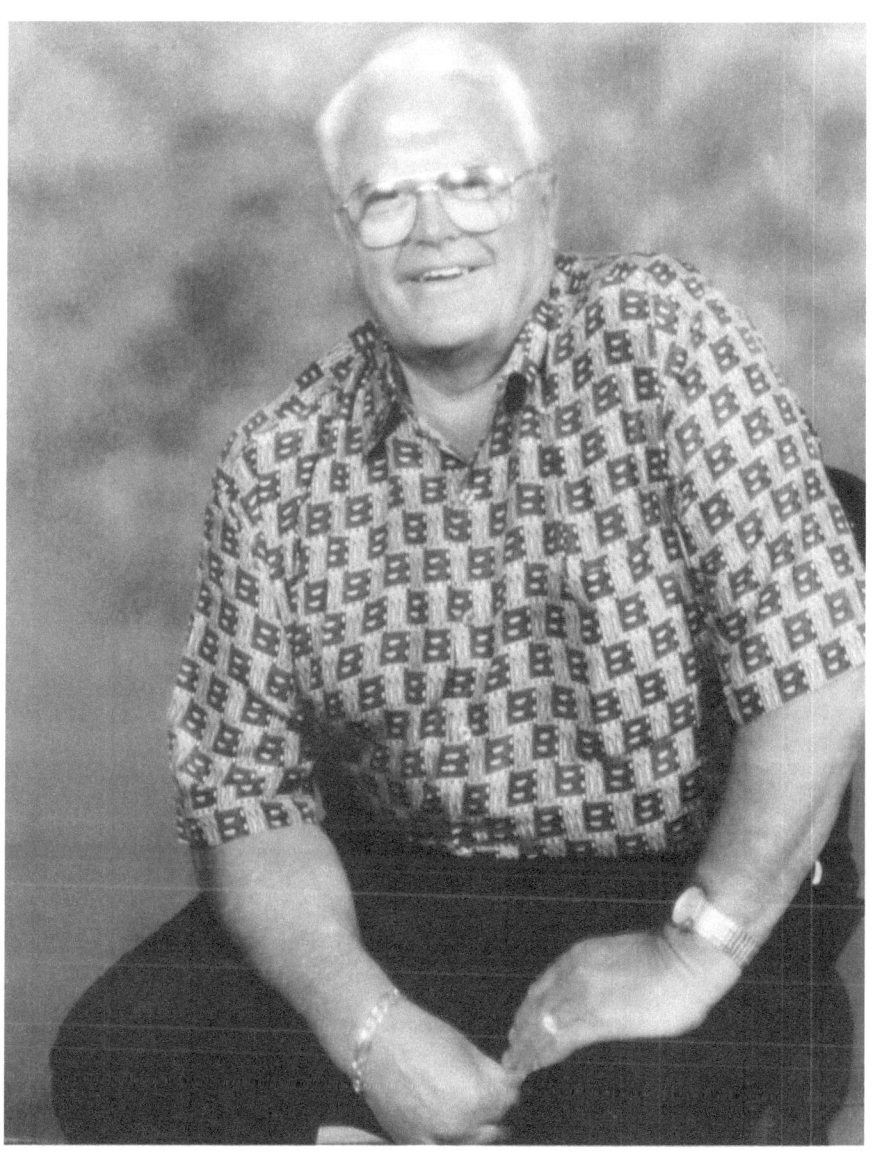

I shall love and miss you always.

Love, Judy

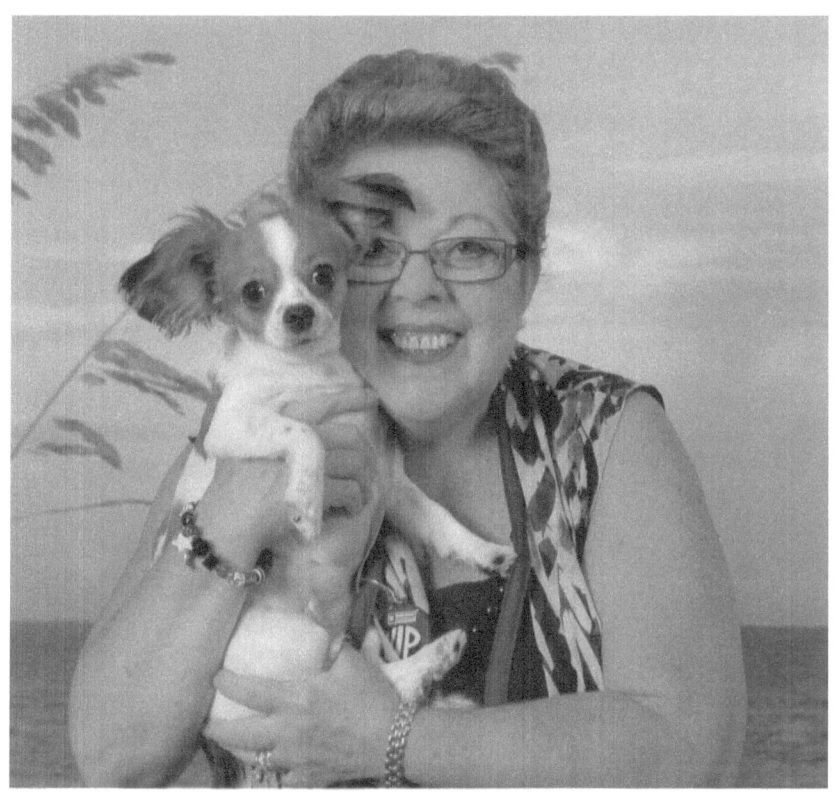

About the Author

Judy Thompson was raised in Brockton, Massachusetts and met her second husband in a widows and widowers support group after her first husband passed away. Following a successful career in real estate, Judy retired in beautiful Tampa Bay. She and her dog, Cuddles, enjoy the views and sunlight of the Florida coastline. Her hobbies include reading, sewing and spending time with her family and friends.